CONTENTS

INTRODUCTION

INTRODUCTION

Welcome to my Change Your Brain Every Day 28-Day Quick-Start Guide. I am so happy that you want to take steps now to make your brain healthier and more vibrant! This program is based on the many valuable lessons we have learned by using brain SPECT imaging to help our patients at Amen Clinics for more than 3 decades. The scans have shown us how daily habits—whether good or bad—have a direct impact on the health and function of each person's brain.

In other words, the choices you make each day can either strengthen your brain and keep it young, or they can lead to mental and physical health issues, increased stress, relationship problems, memory loss, and the rate at which your brain ages.

But the decision is yours! Even if you haven't always been good to your brain, you can make it better by adopting simple, straightforward habits that can change your brain—and your life.

In a short amount of time, this program can help you experience the incredible difference it makes when you choose to love and take care of your brain. I have carefully selected 28 of my favorite brain health strategies and simple daily practices to share with you. They are the same ones I use with my own patients. By incorporating these into your life, you can improve your moods, focus, and energy, sharpen your memory, elevate your mental and physical well-being, and have happier, healthier relationships.

You are not stuck with the brain you have; you can make it better every day. I am grateful to have you join me and the Amen Clinics family in creating a brain health revolution, not only for yourself, but for your loved ones and the generations that follow.

Daniel G. Amen, MD

DAY 1:
IS THIS GOOD FOR MY BRAIN OR BAD FOR MY BRAIN?

This simple question is the mother of all brain-health habits. Building a healthier, more resilient brain and a stronger memory depends on the moment-to-moment, day-to-day decisions you make for yourself. For example:

- When you need a quick pick-me-up, are you going to grab a soda or a cup of green tea?
- If you must drive a short distance into town, will you forego your seatbelt or buckle up?
- After work, are you going to join co-workers for drinks at a bar or meet friends at the gym for a fitness class?

Without consciously thinking about what you are going to do—or not do—unhealthy habits can accumulate to the point that you've compromised not only the health of your body, but of your brain and mental well-being too. That's why, starting today, every time you're about to make a decision for yourself—what you do, what you say, what you eat, and so on—I want you to spend a few seconds and ask yourself this one question:

Is this good for my brain or bad for my brain?

By incorporating this tiny but powerful habit every day, you can make huge strides in your quest to have a healthier brain, and along with it, a better life.

TODAY'S PRACTICE

To practice this habit, in the space below, write down 3 instances when you asked yourself this question, the decision you made, and indicate whether it was good for your brain or bad for it.

Situation	Decision	Good	Bad

DAY 2:
TELL YOUR PREFRONTAL CORTEX WHAT YOU WANT

Your prefrontal cortex (PFC) occupies the front third of your brain. It is the most human and thoughtful part of the brain and is involved with executive functions, including:

- Focus
- Forethought
- Judgment
- Impulse control
- Organization
- Planning
- Empathy
- Learning from the mistakes you make

Because your PFC is intricately tied to so much, it is critical to tell it what you want. To help you do this, we developed a tool called the One Page Miracle (OPM) that we give to all our patients. The OPM will help you stay focused on what you want in the major domains of your life:

- **Biological**—The health of your body and brain
- **Psychological**—Your emotional health and thinking patterns
- **Social**—Your relationships with others, work/school, and finances
- **Spiritual**—Religious or spiritual beliefs, the things you are passionate about, and your connection to past and future generations and the planet.

<><><><><><><><><><><><><><><><> **TODAY'S PRACTICE** <><><><><><><><><><><><><><><><>

Take time today to start filling out your One Page Miracle using the instructions and template on the following pages. Write down what you want—not what you don't want—for each section. Over time, your goals might shift, so update your OPM whenever necessary.

To stay on track with your goals, place your One Page Miracle where you can read it every morning, and then ask yourself:

Does my behavior fit with the goals I have for my life?

One Page Miracle
Instructions

This is the most powerful yet simple motivation tool that can change your life. It is called the **One Page Miracle** because I've seen this exercise quickly focus and change many people's lives.

This exercise encompasses 3 aspects of your life:

1. Core Values: Why do you care? In my clinical practice, I've found that very few people are aware of their own core values, but it's an important piece of the happiness puzzle. It's also important for success too because it helps you focus on what is important to you.

Instructions: Use the Find Your Core Values worksheet on the next page to identify your values then write them in the space provided on the One Page Miracle worksheet on page 6.

2. Purpose: Knowing what your purpose is and what gives your life meaning is critically important to your overall happiness. Research shows that people who are more purposeful have greater happiness and less depression. Plus, they've got more satisfaction, better mental health, personal growth, self-acceptance, longevity—and they sleep better!

Instructions: Use the Know Your Purpose in 5 Questions worksheet on page 5 to identify your purpose and write your answer in the spaces provided on the One Page Miracle worksheet on page 6.

3. Goals: Identifying what you want in each of the Four Circles of your life—Biological, Psychological, Social, and Spiritual—will help guide your thoughts, words, and behaviors. When you tell your brain what you want, your brain will help you make it happen.

Instructions: On the One Page Miracle worksheet, write down your goals—remember to write what you want, not what you don't want—in the spaces provided.

Find Your Core Values

Choose your important characteristics.

Select 1-2 of the following characteristics or traits in each of the Four Circles—Biological, Psychological, Social, and Spiritual—for yourself or your business or organization. Feel free to add your own.

Biological	Psychological	Social	Spiritual
Athleticism	Authenticity	Caring	Acceptance
Beauty	Confidence	Connection	Appreciation
Brain Health	Courage	Dependability	Awareness (Awe)
Energy	Creativity	Empathy	Compassion
Focus	Flexibility	Encouragement	Generosity
Fitness	Forthrightness	Family	Gratitude
Longevity	Fun	Friendships	Growth
Love - Brain/Body	Happiness/Joy	Independence	Humility
Mental clarity	Hard work	Kindness	Inspiration
Physical health	Individuality	Love of others	Love/relationship w/God
Safety	Love-self	Loyalty	Morality
Strength	Open-minded	Outcome driven/service	Patience
Vitality	Positivity	Passion	Prayerful
	Resilience	Significance	Purposeful
	Responsibility	Success	Religious community
	Science-based	Tradition	Surrender
	Security		Transcendence
	Self-control		Wonder

Know Your Purpose in 5 Questions

To discover your purpose, answer the following 5 questions. As an example, look at how influencer Laura Clery answered these questions to help her discover her purpose.

1. What is your name?

Example: Laura Clery

2. What do you love to do? *What do you feel qualified to teach others?*

Example: Create content (comedy) that connects with large groups.

3. Who do you do it for? How does your work connect you to others?

Example: My audience brings me joy.

4. What do others want or need from you?

Example: They want to feel better, more connected, and feel good about themselves.

5. How do they change as a result of what you do?

Example: As a result of what I do, I give people a daily dose of happiness to improve their moods.

Notice that only 2 of the 5 questions are about you; 3 of them are about others. Happiness is found in helping others.

When someone asks, 'What do you do?' answer by telling them your answer to question 5.
Laura's example: *"As a result of what I do, I give people a daily dose of happiness to improve their moods."*

By answering that simple question, you get to share your life's purpose with the many people you meet, which increases dopamine and keeps your pleasure centers healthy.

One Page Miracle Worksheet

Ask yourself if your behavior fits your Core Values, Purpose, and Goals

Core Values

(Insert your important characteristics from the Find Your Core Values worksheet.)

Biological _____

Psychological _____

Social _____

Spiritual _____

Purpose

(Insert your answer to Question #5 on the Know Your Purpose in 5 Questions worksheet.)

_____

Overall Goals

Insert your goals, which are connected to your values, but these are specific to what you want to achieve. For instance, if you choose "Athleticism" as your VALUE, then your GOAL might be to "Run a half marathon in the next 6 months.")

Biological *(Brain & Body)* _____

Psychological *(Mind)* _____

Social *(Relationships, Work, Money)*

- **Relationships**
  - Partner _____
  - Friends _____
  - Family _____
- **Work/School** _____
- **Money** _____

Spiritual *(Meaning & Purpose)*

- **God** _____
- **Planet** _____
- **Connections to Past Generations** _____
- **Connection to Future Generations** _____

Dr. Amen's Recommendations to Help You Reach Your Overall Goals

Biological (*Brain & Body*)

Love your brain and practice the BRIGHT MINDS risk factors (below)

BRIGHT MINDS

B **Blood Flow**
Exercise (walk like you are late for 10,000 steps a day)

R **Retirement/Aging**
Engage in new learning

I **Inflammation**
Eliminate processed foods, floss, take omega-3s and probiotics daily

G **Genetics**
Know and prevent vulnerabilities

H **Head Trauma**
Protect your head

T **Toxins**
Avoid and support 4 organs of detoxification (skin, liver, gut, kidneys)

M **Mental Health**
(see Psychological goals)

I **Immunity/Infections**
Optimize gut & vitamin D levels

N **Neurohormones**
Test and optimize regularly

D **Diabesity**
Maintain healthy weight and blood sugar

S **Sleep**
7-8 hours a night

Social (*Relationships, Work, Money*)

For better connections, practice RELATING:

- Responsibility
- Empathy
- Listening
- Assertiveness
- Time
- Inquire
- Notice what you like
- Grace/forgiveness

Psychological (*Mind*)

Eliminate ANTs (Automatic Negative Thoughts) and write down the negative belief with these five questions.

Ask yourself:

- Is it true?
- Is it absolutely true?
- How do I feel with the thought?
- How do I feel without the thought?
- Is the opposite of the thought true or even truer than the original thought?

Spiritual (*Meaning & Purpose*)

Know your why.

Choose 4-5 anchor images that help you remember what's important to you.

DAY 3:
KNOW YOUR BRAIN TYPE

Have you ever noticed how something that makes you feel content, happy, or energized can cause another person (i.e. your partner or spouse) to feel utterly miserable? The simple reason for this is that not all brains are the same. In fact, there are 16 different brain types—something Amen Clinics discovered through more than 3 decades of using brain SPECT imaging.

Specifically, there are 5 primary brain types:

Brain Type 1: Balanced
Brain Type 2: Spontaneous
Brain Type 3: Persistent
Brain Type 4: Sensitive
Brain Type 5: Cautious

The other 11 types are combinations of types 2-5.

Each brain type has its own preferences, strengths, and vulnerabilities. Thus, knowing your specific brain type helps you understand the ways in which you interact with others and the world around you, as well as what you can do on a daily basis to optimize the health and function of your unique brain.

TODAY'S PRACTICE

To learn what your brain type is, take our free Brain Health Assessment at
brainhealthassessment.com. In the space below, write down your results as well as important characteristics of your brain type.

My brain type is: _____

My brain strengths include: _____

The brain vulnerabilities I want to work on are: _____

_____

DAY 4:
NORMAL IS A MYTH

Many people look outside of themselves and believe that their friends and others are "normal," meaning they don't struggle with any mental health symptoms. If this sounds like your perception, you might be surprised to know that it is very normal for someone to develop mental health symptoms during their lifetime. In fact, most of us have traits from the misfiring of one or more brain systems, which is often the underlying cause of symptoms.

The statistics bear this out. Even before the pandemic hit us, it was known that 51% of the population will have a mental health issue at some point in their life. The most common of these is anxiety, followed closely by depression, ADD/ADHD, addictions, PTSD, and other conditions. Furthermore, 29% of people will have two mental health disorders, and 17% will have three.

So, if you are struggling with any kind of mental health symptoms, you're normal. And contrary to the negative stigma about psychiatric disorders, you are NOT defective or crazy. I want you to know that it's OK to reach out for professional help. Going to a psychiatrist or psychotherapist to work through your issues is a sign of courage and strength—not weakness.

TODAY'S PRACTICE

Below, write down the names of 10 friends. How many of them would benefit by getting help for their mental health issues?

NAME NEEDS HELP?

1. _____

2. _____

3. _____

4. _____

5. _____

6. _____

7. _____

8. _____

9. _____

10. _____

DAY 5:
SUPPLEMENT YOUR BRAIN

If you have a stress-free life; sleep 7-8 hours each night; stay adequately hydrated; have a lifestyle that is free from pollution and toxins; and eat a completely organic, farm-to-table diet; supplements might not be necessary for you. However, most people don't live in that kind of perfect bubble.

Despite an honest effort to be healthy and choose the right foods, many people still have gaps in their nutrition. Therefore, taking basic daily supplements is critical for your health because they can supply the necessary nutrients your body needs, but your diet doesn't fully provide.

I highly recommend that everyone take these 4 supplements daily:

- A high-quality multivitamin
- Omega-3 fatty acids—usually from fish oil, but also available as a vegan product
- A probiotic to support the health of your gut because it is intricately tied to your brain health
- Vitamin D, if necessary to optimize your level

In addition to these daily essentials, certain brain types can benefit from supplements targeted to help balance their brain. For example:

- Spontaneous brains can benefit from a combination of rhodiola, ginseng, green tea extract, ashwagandha, and L-tyrosine.
- Persistent brain types do well with a supplement that has 5HTP and B6 to help boost serotonin.
- Sensitive brains can be sad, so SAMe or a supplement that has saffron, curcumins, and zinc can be helpful.
- Cautious brain types can find a GABA supplement to be calming and help ease stress—this is actually one of Tana's favorites!

TODAY'S PRACTICE

Start your daily supplement regimen today or order the nutraceuticals you need.

DAY 6:
LOVE FOODS THAT LOVE YOU BACK

Food is one of the most important influences on your brain health. Even though your brain is only 2% of your body's weight, it uses 20-30% of the calories you consume, so the quality of what you eat and drink is critical for your mental and physical health. If you mostly eat a fast-food diet, you are much more likely to have brain or mental health issues.

Many children are fed a lot of processed, high-sugar, high-fat foods—think donuts, sweetened cereal, and cookies. They are at the mercy of their parents' and their school system's decisions. Unfortunately, a diet like that can lead to what looks like a learning disorder, ADD/ADHD, or behavior problems as a result of unhealthy nutrition practices. Research studies have shown that when their diet is cleaned up, their symptoms can get better.

And when your diet is improved, your brain will function better too! The good news is that a healthy diet is never about deprivation; it is always about abundance. Fuel your brain with:

- Plenty of fresh produce in a rainbow of colors
- High-quality, lean protein
- Healthy fats, such as coconut, avocado, and olive oils
- Smart carbs that are high in fiber and low in sugar (i.e. quinoa, veggies, and berries)
- Nuts and seeds, especially walnuts and chia and flax seeds because they are high in omega-3s

At the same time, it's important to steer clear of processed high-sugar/high-fat foods, hydrogenated oils, additives, artificial dyes, sugar-laden drinks, alcohol, preservatives—and anything on an ingredient list you cannot pronounce.

TODAY'S PRACTICE

Find 3 breakfasts, 3 lunches, 3 dinners, 3 snacks, and 3 desserts
you love that love you back. Check out the many delicious recipes on brainfitlife.com.
On the following pages you will find more than 100 brain-healthy foods to choose from.

Nuts, Seeds, Nut and Seed Butter, and Meal

- Almond butter
- Almond flour
- Almonds, raw
- Brazil nuts
- Cacao, raw
- Cashews
- Cashew butter
- Chia seeds
- Coconut
- Flax meal
- Flax seeds
- Hemp seeds
- Macadamia nuts
- Oats (whole, gluten-free)
- Pistachios
- Pumpkin seeds
- Quinoa
- Sesame seeds
- Walnuts

Legumes (small amounts, all high in fiber and protein, help balance blood sugar)

- Black beans
- Chickpeas
- Green peas
- Hummus
- Kidney beans
- Lentils
- Navy beans
- Pinto beans

Fruits (choose low-glycemic, high-fiber varieties)

- Acai berries
- Apples
- Avocados
- Blackberries
- Blueberries
- Cantaloupe
- Cherries
- Cranberries
- Figs
- Goji berries
- Goldenberries
- Grapefruit
- Grapes (green)
- Grapes (red)
- Honeydew melon
- Kiwi
- Kumquat
- Lemons
- Lychee
- Mangosteen
- Nectarines
- Olives
- Oranges
- Passion fruit
- Peaches
- Pears
- Plums
- Pomegranates
- Pumpkin
- Raspberries
- Strawberries
- Tangerines
- Tomatoes

Vegetables

- Artichokes
- Arugula
- Asparagus
- Bell peppers
- Beet greens
- Beets
- Broccoli
- Brussels sprouts
- Butter lettuce
- Butternut squash
- Cabbage
- Carrots
- Cauliflower
- Celery
- Celery root
- Chicory
- Chlorella
- Collard greens
- Cucumber
- Eggplant
- Garlic
- Green beans
- Green leaf lettuce
- Horseradish
- Jicama
- Kale
- Leeks
- Maca root
- Mustard greens
- Okra
- Onions
- Parsley
- Parsnips
- Red leaf lettuce
- Romaine lettuce
- Scallions
- Seaweed
- Sea vegetables (including dulse, nori, and spirulina)
- Spinach
- Spirulina
- Summer squash
- Sweet potatoes
- Swiss chard
- Turnips
- Watercress
- Zucchini

Prebiotic Foods

- Artichokes
- Asparagus
- Beans
- Cabbage
- Chia seeds
- Dandelion greens
- Garlic, raw
- Leeks
- Onions
- Psyllium
- Root vegetables (including sweet potatoes, yams, jicama, beets, carrots, and turnips)
- Squash

Probiotic Foods

- Brined vegetables (not pickled with vinegar)
- Chlorella
- Kefir
- Kimchi
- Kombucha tea
- Miso soup
- Pickles
- Sauerkraut (fresh)
- Spirulina

Mushrooms

- Black Truffles
- Chaga
- Chanterelle
- Cordyceps
- Lion's mane
- Maitake
- Oyster
- Porcini
- Reishi
- Shiitake
- Shimeji
- Turkey tail
- White button

Oils

- Avocado oil
- Coconut oil (stable at high temperatures)
- Macadamia nut oil
- Olive oil (stable only at room temperature)

Eggs/Meat/Poultry/Fish

- Ahi
- Arctic char
- Beef (free-range)
- Bison (free-range)
- Chicken
- Eggs (free-range)
- Halibut
- King crab
- Lamb (high in omega-3s)
- Rainbow trout
- Mahi-mahi
- Pork (humanely-raised)
- Salmon (wild-caught)
- Sardines (wild-caught)
- Scallops
- Shrimp
- Tilapia
- Turkey

Herbs and Spices

- Basil
- Black pepper
- Cayenne pepper
- Cinnamon
- Cloves
- Curcumin
- Garlic
- Ginger
- Marjoram

Special Category

- Chocolate (dark, low-sugar)
- Smart mushrooms
- Powdered greens
- Powdered water boost
- Plant-based protein powder
- Shirataki noodles (the root of a wild yam plant—brand name Miracle Noodles—to replace pasta noodles)
- "Zoodles" (zucchini noodles)

Beverages

- Water
- Sparkling water (add a splash of chocolate or orange stevia for a refreshing, calorie-free and toxin-free "soda")
- Spa water (sparkling water with berries, a sprig of mint, or a slice of lemon, orange, peach, or melon)
- Herbal tea
- Green tea
- Unsweetened almond milk (for amazing taste, add a few drops of flavored stevia)
- Unsweetened coconut milk
- Hemp milk
- Coconut water
- Lightly flavored waters, such as Hint
- Vegetable juice or green drinks (without added fruit juice)
- Water with cayenne pepper to boost metabolism
- Beet juice (to increase blood flow)
- Cherry juice (to help sleep)
- Wheatgrass juice

DAY 7:
YOU CANNOT CHANGE WHAT YOU DO NOT MEASURE

Your important health numbers are good indicators of your overall health and how well your body is functioning, so it's crucial to know what they are. If they are out of a healthy range, optimizing them is necessary for bringing your brain, emotions, moods, and body back into balance.

You may already know what some of your health numbers are or can figure them out on your own. For the ones you don't know, ask your doctor to order the appropriate lab tests for you. And if any of the results are outside the healthy range, work with your health care provider to address those issues.

Important Health Numbers to Know:

Body Mass Index (BMI): There are free online programs where you can input your height and weight to determine your BMI. The healthy range is >18.5-24.9.

Waist-to-Height Ratio (WHtR): Measure your waist circumference at the level of your belly button. Divide your waist measurement by your height (in inches). Ideally, it should be 0.5 or less.

Blood Pressure: About 60% of the U.S. population has hypertension or pre-hypertension. As blood pressure increases beyond a healthy level, it lowers blood flow in your brain.

Complete Blood Count (CBC): In addition to identifying important things about your blood, this test can assess for anemia, a condition that is associated with anxiety, insomnia, and fatigue.

C-Reactive Protein: This test measures inflammation in your body, which when elevated, increases your risk for many health and brain problems.

Hemoglobin A1C: Knowing what your blood sugar level is over a period of time is critical, because elevated levels are associated with diabetes and prediabetes, both of which can be harmful to your brain function.

Ferritin: This protein in your blood acts as iron storage, and when it is too low, it can lead to fatigue, symptoms of ADD/ADHD and anxiety as well as sleep problems.

Omega-3 Index: This test measures how much omega-3 EPA/DHA you have in your red blood cells, which ideally should be above 8%. Low omega-3 index numbers can significantly increase the risk of cognitive decline.

Hormone Levels: If your thyroid, testosterone, estrogen, DHEA-S, cortisol, and insulin numbers are not in a healthy range, it can have a direct impact on how your brain is functioning.

Hours You Sleep at Night: Getting less than 7 hours of sleep each night is associated with a number of health issues, not the least of which is developing dementia.

Daily Servings of Fruits and Vegetables: There is a linear correlation between the number of produce servings you have and your degree of happiness. Aim for 8 servings each day.

TODAY'S PRACTICE

In the chart below, fill in your important health numbers for the items you already know, and add the others as soon as you can.

My Tests	My Numbers
Body Mass Index (BMI)	
Waist-to-Height Ratio (WHtR)	
Blood Pressure	
Complete Blood Count (CBC) abnormalities (if any):	
C-Reactive Protein	
Hemoglobin A1C	
Ferritin	
Vitamin D	
Omega-3 Index	
Hormone Levels:	
Cortisol	
DHEA-S	
Estrogen	
Insulin	
Testosterone	
Thyroid	
Hours of Sleep at Night	
Daily Servings of Fruits and Vegetables	

DAY 8:
YOUR BRAIN IS A SNEAKY ORGAN

Everyone has weird, stupid, or unsavory thoughts, but people with good frontal lobe function don't blurt them out. Why is that? Your frontal lobes are like having a personal CEO, that in addition to helping with planning, judgment, and forethought, controls your "brakes" and the urge to do something impulsively. In other words, you keep your mouth shut when it's in your best interest to do so, and you show up when you're supposed to. Simple behaviors like these are a reflection of frontal lobes that work well, which in turn is linked to greater success, health, and longevity.

To that point, a longitudinal study conducted at Stanford University on personality traits that began in 1921 with more than 1,500 10-year-old kids, followed them throughout their lives. Interestingly, the outcome of this research found that the key to living a longer life wasn't happiness, coming from a wealthy family, partying, or having a big group of friends—it was their level of conscientiousness.

So, just as you wouldn't give in to a child every time they throw a tantrum, it's important that you don't give in to your own unhealthy impulses, such as:

- Not following through on a commitment
- Saying something unkind to someone when you're feeling cranky
- Downing a pint of your favorite ice cream just because it tastes good

To keep your brain healthy and fortify your frontal lobe function, you need to practice saying "no" to yourself rather than caving into behaviors that will cause you more problems. Impulse control and conscientiousness are so important!

TODAY'S PRACTICE

Don't say everything you think. Work on inhibiting your unhealthy impulses.

DAY 9:
BRIGHT MINDS – B IS FOR BLOOD FLOW

If you want to keep your brain healthy or rescue it if it's in trouble, you have to prevent or treat the 11 major risk factors that can steal your mind. BRIGHT MINDS is an acronym we developed that represents each of the risk factors that can hurt your brain and diminish your memory. Today, I am going to tell you about the first one—B—which stands for blood flow.

Your blood flow supplies all the cells in your body and brain with oxygen and vital nutrients needed for survival. Having healthy blood vessels is critical for this process. However, there are many things that can decrease blood flow and increase your risk for memory problems. In fact, low blood flow is the #1 brain imaging predictor of Alzheimer's disease. Therefore, it is imperative to protect the health of your blood vessels.

Behaviors and conditions that hurt your blood flow. Check any that apply to you:

- Smoking, vaping, or chewing tobacco—using nicotine in any form
- Lack of exercise
- Drinking too much alcohol
- Marijuana
- The Standard American Diet (SAD)—i.e. high-sugar, high-fat, and processed foods
- Hypertension and heart disease
- High cholesterol
- Substance abuse
- Erectile dysfunction

Your blood vessels are systemic, so whatever hurts your heart, also hurts your brain and your genitals.

TODAY'S PRACTICE

Boost your blood flow by incorporating these 3 things into your lifestyle:

- Eat more beets.
- Exercise regularly.
- Take a gingko biloba supplement.

The older you get, the more serious you need to be about brain health. Advancing in your years is the #1 risk factor for memory problems and developing some type of dementia. The scary reality is that half of all people aged 85 and older will be diagnosed with Alzheimer's disease. But getting older does not mean your cognitive function has to decline; however, when you stop learning, your brain starts dying.

If you are retired and spend a lot of time in a recliner watching TV, you are not doing yourself any favors because you are promoting your own aging. If you want to keep your brain healthy and memory strong, it is important that you stay mentally and socially active. From the list below, identify any risk factors that apply to you:

Retirement/Aging Risk Factors

- Age
- Retired
- Don't engage in learning new things
- Social isolation

- Elevated or low iron level
- Shortened telomeres—the casings on the end of your chromosomes (determined by a blood test)

The best way to counteract any of these risks is to regularly challenge yourself by doing or learning new things that interest you, such as:

- Take a class to learn something new
- Learn to play a musical instrument
- Volunteer for an organization you like and meet new people
- Challenge yourself by developing new skills
- Join a fitness class for weight training. The stronger you are the less likely you will be to get Alzheimer's disease!

And if your iron (ferritin) level is too high or too low, work with your health care provider to get it into the healthy range.

TODAY'S PRACTICE

Find something new to learn and spend at least 15 minutes a day working on it.

DAY 11:
BRIGHT MINDS—I IS FOR INFLAMMATION

When you have inflammation in your body, it's like a fire alarm going off trying to tell you that something is wrong. Whatever it is, your immune system rushes white blood cells to fight "the invader." We have seen this a lot with COVID-19 infections—the inflammation goes to the brain. We even saw these changes on brain images of patients who had previously been scanned but developed other symptoms after getting COVID. Their new scans showed areas of dramatically increased activity because of the inflammation. But that's not the only thing that causes it.

As a whole, we are a physically inflamed society for a number of reasons, including:

- The excess intake of sugar and processed foods
- Gum disease, which is linked to heart disease and brain problems
- Increases in autoimmune disorders that cause the body to fight against itself
- Gut health issues. (If your gut isn't healthy, your brain is not going to be healthy either because 92% of your body's serotonin is produced in your gut.)

We believe one of the biggest culprits of gut problems is related to eating gluten. While about 7% of the population has obvious gluten sensitivity, the rest of us can still be causing damage to our body by consuming it, such as developing leaky gut.

TODAY'S PRACTICE

- Start flossing every day if you aren't already doing so.
- Take a daily probiotic to support your gut health.
- Eat foods high in omega-3 fatty acids (they are anti-inflammatory), such as walnuts, chia and flax seeds, and cold-water fatty fish like salmon. And take an omega-3 supplement that has 1,400 to 2,800 mg a day in roughly a 60/40 EPA:DHA ratio.

Everyone has genetic inheritances related to physical or mental health issues, but just because you carry a certain gene, in most cases, it doesn't necessarily mean you will develop the condition. This is so important to understand. Your genes tell you what your vulnerabilities are. I often say that, metaphorically, genes load the gun, but it is behavior that pulls the trigger—or not.

In addition to that, the neuroscience field of epigenetics has discovered that your habits can turn on or turn off the genes that make illness more or less likely to manifest, not only in you, but also in your children and the generations that follow. Your lifestyle choices can make a huge difference in whether or not a gene gets passed along.

For example, I have a family history of obesity and heart disease, but I am neither overweight nor struggling with heart problems. My wife Tana comes from a long line of women who experienced trauma. She also endured childhood trauma that resulted in depression and anxiety at times in her life. She did not want to pass along these problems to her own daughter.

You can make the decision to take responsibility for how you respond to your genetic risks, too. This is critical, especially for anyone who has a family history of memory problems, Alzheimer's disease, or another type of dementia. If you carry 1 or 2 copies of the APOE4 gene or presenilin genes, you must take your brain health very seriously.

TODAY'S PRACTICE

- Know your family history and write down any mental health or memory issues among your relatives. _____

  _____

- Talk to your health care provider about any recommended screenings or blood tests, then write down any genetic vulnerabilities here: _____

  _____

- Begin a prevention program to minimize your genetic risk(s). Write down 1 thing you will start today: _____

  _____

DAY 13:
BRIGHT MINDS—H IS FOR HEAD TRAUMA

Your brain controls everything you do, think, say, feel, and desire, but your brain is very soft—its consistency is somewhere between egg whites and Jell-O. Therefore, if you hit your head, you can damage your brain and cause a multitude of symptoms. Having used SPECT imaging to look at the brain for more than 3 decades, we know that even mild traumatic brain injuries are a major cause of psychiatric problems. Unfortunately, many mental health professionals don't understand this because they don't look at their patients' brains.

Most people think of head trauma as a cracked skull resulting in a loss of consciousness, but brain injuries can also be caused by much less serious events. When asked, many of our patients don't even remember that they ever had a brain injury, so we have to ask multiple times, in multiple ways. For example:

- Did you ever fall out of a tree or off the monkey bars?

- Did you play contact sports like football or hit soccer balls with your head?

- Have you ever been in a motor vehicle accident or gotten whiplash?

- Have you ever been hit in the head with something that made you see stars or feel dizzy?

Other than when a person is diagnosed with a concussion, most people tend to shake off an impact to their head and forget about it. However, the brain's delicate texture makes it very susceptible to injury.

And children are especially vulnerable because the human brain isn't fully developed until our mid-twenties, so if you have kids, it's critical to protect their brains. Don't let them do headers at soccer, make sure they wear a helmet when biking or skateboarding, and so on.

TODAY'S PRACTICE

Stop texting while you are driving or walking to lower the risk of hitting your head.

DAY 14:
BRIGHT MINDS—T IS FOR TOXINS

Toxins seem to be everywhere in the environment and are linked to all sorts of health issues, including brain problems and dementia. They can be inhaled, such as with air pollution and cigarette smoke, ingested through what you eat and drink, or absorbed through your skin.

There are so many things that are toxic to your brain and body! Some of the more obvious ones are:

- Recreational drugs and alcohol
- Medications like Xanax and opiates
- Anesthesia
- Mold inside the walls of your home
- Pesticides in the food you eat

But there are also less well-known sources of toxins, such as the skin-care products you put on your body that contain parabens and phthalates. These can include lotions, sunscreen, fragrances, and other personal products.

Because of the ubiquity of toxins all around us, it is important to support the 4 organs of detoxification: your liver, kidneys, gut, and skin. Here's how:

- Avoid anything that's potentially toxic for you.
- Drink more water to flush things out through your kidneys.
- Eat more fiber to flush things out through your gut.
- Eat healthy foods that support your intestinal flora.
- Avoid alcohol and the recreational use of drugs.
- Eat more detoxifying vegetables like brassicas—Brussels sprouts, cauliflower, kale, broccoli, and cabbage.
- Regularly break a sweat with exercise and by taking saunas.

TODAY'S PRACTICE

- Support your 4 organs of detoxification by incorporating at least 1 of the suggestions above today.
- Choose 1 room in your home—such as the kitchen, bathroom, or garage—and read the product labels to identify any toxic ingredients.
- Download an app like THINK DIRTY and use it to scan your personal products to see how toxic they are to your body.

DAY 15:
BRIGHT MINDS—M IS FOR MENTAL HEALTH

Mental health issues such as depression, ADD/ADHD, bipolar disorder, PTSD, anxiety, chronic stress, and a history of childhood trauma can increase the risk for memory issues, heart disease, cancer, and other health problems. Therefore, it is important to address any mental health symptoms you have as soon as possible. Not only can treatment make you feel better, but it can also help protect the health of your body and brain.

This is especially important if you endured chaos, neglect, abuse, or other traumas during childhood, because it may have put you at an elevated risk for significant health problems.

What are referred to as Adverse Childhood Experiences—or ACEs—often result in a young person being exposed to toxic stress which increases the risk for developing 7 of the 10 leading causes of death, including cancer.

The ACE Questionnaire covers the major sources of childhood trauma, including:

- Emotional, physical, and sexual abuse
- Neglect
- Household substance abuse and/or mental illness
- Domestic violence
- Incarceration of any household members

The scoring range is 0 to 10, and a score greater than 4 is believed to increase the risk for health problems as a result of the toxic stress experienced during childhood.

TODAY'S PRACTICE

Take the ACE Questionnaire on the following page to determine your score and enter it here:

My ACE Score is_____

Adverse Childhood Experiences (ACEs) Questionnaire

To determine how many ACEs you had, put a checkmark next to any item in the questionnaire below that applies to you. Then add up the checkmarks to get your ACE score.

☐ 1. Before your 18th birthday, did a parent or other adult in the household often or very often: swear at you, insult you, put you down, or humiliate you? OR act in a way that made you afraid that you might be physically hurt?

☐ 2. Before your 18th birthday, did a parent or other adult in the household often or very often: push, grab, slap, or throw something at you? OR ever hit you so hard that you had marks or were injured?

☐ 3. Before your 18th birthday, did an adult or person at least five years older than you ever: touch or fondle you or have you touch their body in a sexual way? OR attempt to or have oral, anal, or vaginal intercourse with you?

☐ 4. Before your 18th birthday, did you often or very often feel that: no one in your family loved you or thought you were important or special? OR your family didn't look out for each other, feel close to each other, or support each other?

☐ 5. Before your 18th birthday, did you often or very often feel that: you didn't have enough to eat, had to wear dirty clothes, and had no one to protect you? OR your parents were too drunk or high to take care of you or take you to the doctor if you needed it?

☐ 6. Before your 18th birthday, was a biological parent ever lost to you through divorce, abandonment, or other reason?

☐ 7. Before your 18th birthday, was your mother or stepmother: often or very often pushed, grabbed, slapped, or had something thrown at her? OR sometimes, often, or very often kicked, bitten, hit with a fist, or hit with something hard? OR ever repeatedly hit for at least a few minutes or threatened with a gun or knife?

☐ 8. Before your 18th birthday, did you live with anyone who was a problem drinker or alcoholic, or who used street drugs?

☐ 9. Before your 18th birthday, was a household member depressed or mentally ill, or did a household member attempt suicide?

☐ 10. Before your 18th birthday, did a household member go to prison?

DAY 16:
BRIGHT MINDS—I IS FOR IMMUNITY AND INFECTIONS

Infectious diseases don't just affect the health of your body, they can affect your brain too. During the last decade or so much has been discovered about the impact a condition like Lyme disease has on mental health, and recently, it has become quite evident that COVID-19 can adversely affect the brain too. At Amen Clinics, we have seen increased numbers of patients with depression, anxiety, and even psychosis, and 80% of patients who had COVID-19 developed memory and focus problems.

The best defense against any type of infection is having a strong immune system, and there are some simple things you can do to bolster yours. For one, it's important to check your vitamin D level and if it's not in the healthy range (50-100 mg/dL), you'll want to optimize it. Another way to bolster your health is by including these immune-boosting foods in your diet:

- Onions
- Garlic
- Mushrooms, especially Lion's mane, reishi, cordyceps, and turkey tail
- Ginger—put some in lemon water
- Saffron—add to a meal or a cup of tea

The same strategy that this 28-Day Quick-Start Guide started with, "Is this good for my brain or bad for it," also applies to your body. If you have been struggling with symptoms for a while and aren't getting well, consider working with a functional medicine doctor to be tested for an underlying infection. This can be really helpful for anyone who has an autoimmune disorder. In these conditions, the immune system is overactive and attacks itself, almost as though it sees the person's body as the problem. While the symptoms can tell you what kind of disorder it is, it does not tell you why it is occurring.

Through decades of experience, the doctors at Amen Clinics have treated many patients whose fatigue, mental health struggles, and cognitive issues were caused by an underlying, but previously undetected, infection. With the right treatment plan, the patients found significant relief from their symptoms

TODAY'S PRACTICE

- Get your vitamin D level checked and optimize it if necessary.
- Start adding more garlic, onions, mushrooms, ginger, and saffron to your diet.

Your hormones control many of the basic functions in your body and have a tremendous impact on how you feel physically and mentally. Your brain is also involved in this process, signaling the release of hormones, and being influenced by the various hormones in your body.

These tiny chemical messengers work together in a delicate balance, which, when disrupted by too little or too much of any one of them, can have a negative effect on your behavior, emotions, energy, or the way you think. When your neurohormones—the hormones that affect your brain are out of balance, it can impact brain function and lead to symptoms of depression, anxiety, fatigue, irritation, memory problems, anger, and more as well as lead to an increased risk of heart disease, diabetes, Alzheimer's disease, and certain types of cancer.

- **Cortisol**—helps to manage stress and anxiety
- **DHEA-S**—fights stress and depression, decreases brain inflammation
- **Estrogen and Progesterone**—when balanced, promote stable moods
- **Insulin**—balances blood sugar
- **Testosterone**—affects mood, motivation, sexuality, and strength
- **Thyroid**—regulates energy and mood

Aside from natural aging processes or women's monthly menstrual cycles, there are a number of ways your neurohormones can get out of whack. They can be disrupted by inflammation, a high-sugar diet, head injuries, smoking, processed foods, obesity, unhealthy fats, wheat, pesticides and other environmental toxins, leaky gut syndrome, chronic stress, vitamin deficiencies, and more.

TODAY'S PRACTICE

- Avoid neurohormone disruptors.
- If you haven't already done so, schedule an appointment to have your neurohormone levels tested.

DAY 18:
BRIGHT MINDS—D IS FOR DIABESITY

The word diabesity is a combination of being obese (or overweight) and/or having high blood sugar levels and being diabetic or prediabetic. If your weight is unhealthy or blood sugar is out of balance, it is a disaster for your brain function. In fact, Amen Clinics has published 3 research studies that found as the weight of a person goes up, the size and function of their brain goes down.

This problem has become an epidemic in the U.S. that continues to get worse:

- 70% of people are considered to be overweight, and 40% are obese.
- Approximately 14% of the population has diabetes, and another 36% are prediabetic.

Not only does diabesity increase the risk for more illnesses, but it is also one of the main reasons for the increase of mental health and brain health issues in people of all ages. Being overweight/obese can elevate your chances of developing diabetes, a medical problem that causes damage to the blood vessels throughout your body and brain. This in turn can lead to other serious conditions, including hypertension, heart disease, stroke, vascular dementia, and Alzheimer's disease.

If you are affected by diabesity you can take steps now to reclaim your health. One of the most important ways to do this is by switching to a healthier diet and choosing foods you love that love you back, like I talked about earlier. It's also important to pay attention to the number of calories you eat, not so you become skinny, but to get to a weight that is healthy for you.

The good news is that if you're eating high-quality calories, like lots of fresh produce and clean protein, you can actually eat more food than, for example, the high-glycemic, low-fiber, processed foods that many people get addicted to and are fundamental causes of obesity and type 2 diabetes.

TODAY'S PRACTICE

- Stop loving foods that harm you. Instead, choose to love foods that love you back.
- Weigh yourself at the same time every day.
- If you are trying to lose weight, write down everything you eat so you can keep track of how many calories you are consuming each day.

Sleep is such a vital component of good health, yet 60 million people in the U.S. have sleep problems. When you are asleep, your brain cleanses itself of toxins and cellular debris that accumulate during the day. It also consolidates memory and learning and prepares for the next day. The complex processes that occur while you sleep are also very important for neurotransmitter production, appetite control, and the health of your immune system.

Because of this, it is crucial to get at least 7 hours of good quality sleep each night. Unfortunately, there are many things that interfere with getting the right amount of shut-eye to keep your brain and body healthy.

Some of the most common sleep stealers include:

- Caffeine, especially later in the day

- Eating too close to bedtime

- A bedroom that is too warm or too noisy

- Difficulty turning off your worries at night

- Hormonal imbalances or other medical issues

- Shift work

- Depression or anxiety

- Untreated sleep apnea—Do you snore or stop breathing multiple times at night?

Are any of these hurting your sleep?

If you are tired during the day due to inadequate or unrestorative sleep, improving your sleep hygiene can make a huge difference in protecting the health of your brain and body.

◇◇◇◇◇◇◇◇◇◇◇◇◇◇◇◇◇◇◇◇◇◇◇ **TODAY'S PRACTICE** ◇◇◇◇◇◇◇◇◇◇◇◇◇◇◇◇◇◇◇◇◇◇◇

Avoid anything that hurts your sleep and do the things that help you get 7-8 hours of sleep each night. Here are our 20 favorite strategies to help you get the zzzzzz's you need. Choose 1 of them to try tonight.

1. Keep your bedroom cool.
2. Make your bedroom completely dark or wear an eye mask
3. Turn off phones and other gadgets by the bed, or at least turn off the sound.
4. Make your bedroom noise-free or wear ear plugs.
5. Try to fix emotional problems before getting in bed with a positive text, email, or intention to deal with the issues tomorrow. If your thoughts are stuck in a loop, use your journal to write down your concerns, what you can do about the situation, and what is out of your control.
6. Maintain a regular sleep schedule—going to bed at the same time each night and waking up at the same time each day, including on weekends. In addition, get up at the same time each day regardless of sleep duration the previous night.
7. Don't allow pets in your bedroom or at least keep them off the bed.
8. Create a soothing nighttime routine that encourages sleep. A warm bath, meditation, or massage can help you relax.
9. Some people like to read themselves to sleep. If that's what you do, don't read an action-packed thriller or a horror story—they aren't likely to help you drift off to sleep.
10. Sound therapy can induce a very peaceful mood and lull you to sleep. Consider soothing nature sounds, wind chimes, a fan, or soft music. You can find sleep-enhancing music by Grammy award winning producer, Barry Goldstein, on *mybrainfitlife.com*.
11. Drink a mixture of warm unsweetened almond milk, a teaspoon of vanilla (the real stuff, not imitation), and a few drops of stevia. This may increase serotonin in your brain and help you sleep.
12. Take a warm bath or shower before bed.
13. Wear socks to bed. Researchers have found that warm hands and feet were the best predictor of rapid sleep onset.
14. If you wake up in the middle of the night, refrain from looking at the clock. Checking the time can make you feel anxious, which aggravates the problem.
15. Use the bed and bedroom only for sleep or sex. Sexual activity releases many natural hormones, releases muscle tension, and boosts a sense of well-being. Adults with healthy sex lives tend to sleep better.
16. Talk to your doctor if you're taking any medications that can disrupt sleep, such as asthma medications, antihistamines, cough medicines, anticonvulsants, or stimulants prescribed for ADD/ADHD.
17. When you go to bed, ask yourself, "What went well today?" This will help set you up for more pleasant dreams and better sleep.
18. Hypnosis or meditation can help. We have audio downloads on *mybrainfitlife.com* that can be helpful.
19. Use the scent of lavender to enhance sleep. It has been shown to decrease anxiety and improve mood and sleep.
20. Natural supplements, such as a combination of melatonin, magnesium, and GABA may be helpful.

DAY 20:
KNOW YOUR DRAGONS

Our colleague, Sharon May, introduced us to the concept of Dragons from the Past, which are the big emotional issues each of us has that are always "breathing fire" on the emotional part of our brain. All of us have these internal dragons. Not only can they cause us distress, especially when we aren't aware of them, but they can also interfere with our relationships too.

In my book, *Your Brain is Always Listening*, I write extensively about the 13 Dragons from the Past, and I describe the origins of each dragon, how they get triggered, and what reactions they can cause you to have as well as straightforward steps to tame them.

Here's a quick overview of the 13 Dragons from the Past:

1. Abandoned, Invisible, or Insignificant Dragons—feel alone, unseen, or unimportant
2. Inferior or Flawed Dragons—feel inferior to others
3. Anxious Dragons—feel fearful and overwhelmed
4. Wounded Dragons—bruised by past trauma
5. Should and Shaming Dragons—racked with guilt
6. Special, Spoiled, or Entitled Dragons—feel more special than others
7. Responsible Dragons—need to take care of others
8. Angry Dragons—harbor hurts and rage
9. Judgmental Dragons—hold harsh or critical opinions of others due to past injustices
10. Death Dragons—fear the future and lack of a meaningful life
11. Grief and Loss Dragons—feel loss and/or have a fear of loss
12. Hopeless or Helpless Dragons—have a pervasive sense of despair and discouragement
13. Ancestral Dragons—affected by issues from past generations

Individuals who have a high ACE (Adverse Childhood Experiences) score tend to have a lot of dragons because of the early adversity in their lives. Being aware of which dragons you have and using the right strategies can help you overcome them.

TODAY'S PRACTICE

Take the Know Your Dragons quiz at *KnowYourDragons.com* to discover which ones you have, how they affect you, and what you can do about them.

DAY 21:
HOW TO BREAK AN ANXIETY ATTACK IN 2 MINUTES

Getting anxious when you are in a stressful situation is normal, but sometimes that anxiety can get overwhelming, giving you the urge to run away. While it is appropriate to flee if you are concerned about your safety, most other situations are not life-threatening. They just fill you with dread, such as having to do an important interview or other nerve-racking situations that make you break a sweat and feel like your mind has gone blank.

Fortunately, there are a few simple things you can do to quickly break an anxiety attack, calm your nerves, and regain your mental acuity.

1. First, do not leave the situation unless you are in real danger. Staying put helps you overcome your initial "fight-or-flight" response and tells your brain there is no reason to flee. If you do leave, that situation will have control over you, and you may never again risk doing whatever it is for fear of having another anxiety attack.

2. The second thing to do is breathe deeply using diaphragmatic breathing. Rather than take rapid breaths from your upper chest (which makes you feel more anxious), breathe with your belly. When you inhale, your belly should push out, and when you exhale, it should move in toward your spine. Breathe in this specific pattern:

    •   Inhale for 4 seconds

    •   Hold for a second

    •   Exhale for 8 seconds

    •   Hold for a second

    •   Repeat. Within 3 of these deep breaths, you will feel calmer.

3. Next, write down what you are thinking because that is what is making you so anxious.

TODAY'S PRACTICE

Do some diaphragmatic breathing for a few minutes today—and every day—to help you manage anxious feelings.

It's not the thoughts you have that make you suffer. It's the thoughts you attach to that make you suffer. Your thoughts come from all sorts of places. They can get written into your genetic code. They come from the voices of your parents, siblings, friends, and coworkers. They come from the news you watch, the music you listen to, the experiences you have, and so on.

Just because you have a thought has nothing to do with whether or not it's true, and whether or not it's helping you. And if you don't learn to direct your thoughts, they'll control you and hurt you. This is why I want to share with you my favorite technique for getting control over your automatic negative thoughts (ANTs).

How to Kill the ANTs:

Whenever you feel mad, sad, nervous, or out of control, write down the automatic negative thought—the ANT— that is causing you distress. Then ask yourself these 5 questions about that thought:

1. Is it true?

2. Is it absolutely true, with 100% certainty?

3. How do I feel when I believe this thought?

4. How would I feel if I didn't have this thought?

5. Next, turn the ANT around to its exact opposite, and ask yourself if the opposite thought is true or even truer than the original thought. Then write down 3 examples of why this new thought is more accurate than the ANT.

TODAY'S PRACTICE

Using this Kill the ANTs strategy, challenge at least 1 of your ANTs today. Start keeping a log of your ANTs and work on each one until you have exterminated all of them.

1. Is it true? _____

2. Is it absolutely true, with 100% certainty? _____

3. How do I feel when I believe this thought? _____

4. How would I feel if I didn't have this thought? _____

5. Next, turn the ANT around to its exact opposite. Is this thought true or truer than the original thought? _____

Write down 3 examples of why this new thought is more accurate than the ANT.

_____

_____

_____

DAY 23:
POSITIVITY BIAS TRAINING

Our brains are naturally wired for negativity. Back in the caveman days, it helped our ancestors survive, knowing that at any moment a large creature could eat them for breakfast, lunch, or dinner; thus, they needed anxiety to keep them alert. A similar thing happens to people who have experienced trauma. Many of the anxious, stressed, and depressed patients we see at Amen Clinics have a strong negativity bias.

You can suffer less by shifting your brain to be more positive—not in a Pollyanna kind of way—but by training your brain to look for what is right, rather than what is wrong. Even on your most challenging days, this is something you can do by incorporating these 3 simple habits that, within a few weeks, can help you feel happier and less burdened by depressive and/or anxious thoughts.

1. Begin every day by saying, "Today is going to be a great day." By doing this, your brain will begin to view the day from a positive perspective, rather than a negative one.

2. End each day by asking yourself, "What went well today?" You might at first recall the more notable events, but as you keep thinking, other things you might have glossed over will pop into your mind. After 3 weeks of doing this every day, you'll increase your level of happiness.

3. Pay attention to the daily micro-moments of happiness—the little things that lift you up, make you smile, or invoke a little sense of awe. Whatever gives you a moment of joy in some way, take note of it.

TODAY'S PRACTICE

- Every morning, say, "Today is going to be a great day."
- End each day by asking yourself, "What went well today?"
- Write down 5 of your micro-moments of happiness from today.

MY MICRO-MOMENTS OF HAPPINESS

1._____
2._____
3._____
4._____
5._____

DAY 24:
EMDR FOR PAST TRAUMA AND TO CALM ANXIETY

One of the most successful therapies for helping people work through past traumas is known as EMDR, which stands for eye movement desensitization and reprocessing. It was developed in the 1980s by a psychologist named Francine Shapiro, who noticed that when she was out walking and looked to the left, then to the right, whatever was bothering her seemed to bother her less.

EMDR incorporates alternating hemispheric brain stimulation by using back and forth eye movements, tapping on the knees, hand-held pulsating devices, or headphones. This reduces the emotional charge of traumatic memories and helps them become "unstuck" in the brain so that they can be reprocessed from a more present state. This therapy helps the intensity of a bad memory or experience dissipate so you don't keep getting triggered (consciously or unconsciously) by recollections, smells, sounds, images, or feelings that remind you of what happened.

Although EMDR is most well-known for treating trauma and PTSD, it can also be very helpful for other conditions, including anxiety, grief and loss, addictions, depression, eating disorders, phobias, and others.

TODAY'S PRACTICE

Visit emdria.org to learn more about how EMDR can help you.

DAY 25:
RELATING

If you are struggling to get along with the people you love, adopt and practice the foundational habits of RELATING to increase your chances of having better relationships.

R-E-L-A-T-I-N-G

- **R** is for Responsibility: Rather than playing the blame game, take responsibility for your relationships. When you pretend you are helpless in the relationship, you give your spouse/significant other total control, which then fuels resentment, distress, anxiety, depression, and feeling hopeless.

- **E** is for Empathy: Mirror neurons in our brain allow us to "read" one another and mimic certain actions (like yawning), thus help us to experience feelings of empathy and compassion for others. This is important when your loved one has a brain type that is different than yours. Learn what makes them happy or unhappy and try to see things through their eyes.

- **L** is for Listening: Even when 2 people love each other, if their communication skills are poor, it can spell doom. Therefore, it is essential to communicate well with each other if you want to build and maintain a strong relationship. This means don't interrupt or finish your spouse's thoughts or be thinking about what you want to say rather than listening to what is being said.

- **A** is for Assertiveness: When you express your feelings and thoughts in a firm yet reasonable way, say no when you want to, and don't let others emotionally run over you, you are being assertive. Staying in control of yourself, not giving in to the anger of another person, and sticking up for what you believe is right, are signs of healthy assertiveness.

- **T** is for Time: There is no getting around having "special time" together if you want your relationship to flourish. It's critical that you schedule time during which you can focus on each other without distractions. Go on dates, spend time in the outdoors, and do things you both enjoy. Whatever it is, turn off your cell phones and be present with one another.

- **I** is for Inquiry: People can get so wrapped up in their negative thoughts that they inadvertently sabotage their relationships. But you can break this destructive habit. Whenever you have an automatic negative thought (ANT) about your relationship that makes you upset, write it down and ask yourself the 5 questions I described earlier.

- **N** Is for Noticing What You Like a Lot More Than What You Don't Like: This practice is known as positive reinforcement—and it's one of our favorites because it really works. In fact, married couples who give each other 5 times more positive comments than negative ones are significantly less likely to get divorced.

- **G** is for Grace: An unwillingness to forgive others is associated with higher levels of stress and it adversely affects mental and physical health. Learning to forgive and offer grace in a relationship can be powerfully healing and plays a vital role in helping a relationship flourish.

TODAY'S PRACTICE

Throughout the day, notice what you like about others more than what you don't like and write it down below.

WHAT I LIKE ABOUT OTHERS

1._____

2._____

3._____

4._____

5._____

DAY 26:
ACTIVE LISTENING

As I mentioned when I talked about the L in RELATING (which stands for listening), good communication skills are critical for healthy relationships. Being a good listener is so important that I want to re-emphasize it by focusing on active listening today.

Feeling heard and hearing others—whether it's your partner, co-worker, friend, or child— facilitates trust, understanding, and bonding between people, and are essential components of communication in all relationships.

The problem is, not everyone is very good at it. Fortunately, you can learn to be better at paying attention to others by learning and practicing the following techniques.

7 Active Listening Skills:

1. Minimize distractions (i.e. put down your phone).

2. Be present. Smile, nod silently, lean in, or say "I see," "I understand," "Uh-huh," or "Hmmm."

3. Make eye contact.

4. Don't interrupt the other person. Sometimes people worry that they will forget what they want to say, so they interrupt. When that happens the person speaking can lose their train of thought, and the conversation goes in a completely different direction.

5. Don't judge, because when you do, it stops the conversation or leads to an argument.

6. Give the person some space and allow for periods of silence, rather than filling up every second with talking. Be patient and let them take their time.

7. Repeat back what has been said and listen for the feelings behind the words. When you are dismissive about what a person is saying, you diminish their feelings.

TODAY'S PRACTICE

Practice active listening today—and every day.

DAY 27:
THE FORK IN THE ROAD EXERCISE

Brain health is a choice you get to make every day of your life, but I know it isn't always easy to remember this. And without keeping it in the forefront of your mind, you might be vulnerable to falling back into old habits, even though you know they don't serve you well.

To help you continue working on having a better brain every day, I want you to do one of our favorite motivational exercises called The Fork in the Road.

Vividly imagine you are out in the countryside and see a fork in the road that has two paths. Imagine that the fork on the left leads to a future of pain. It's a future in which you don't care about your brain and continue to do the unhealthy things you've always done. What will your life be like in a year? In 5 years? And in 10, 20, or even 30 years? Imagine your brain rapidly aging because of your lifestyle choices and the brain fog, low energy, depression, weight gain, memory loss, and physical illness that go along with those problems.

Now, imagine that the fork on the right is a future of health—one in which you care about your brain and practice brain health every day. What will your life be like in a year? In 5, 10, 20, or 30 years? I want you to imagine your brain getting healthier and younger and all that goes with that: a brighter mood, mental clarity, better energy, a great memory, a trimmer and healthier body, more vitality, and a younger brain.

With this knowledge, it's your decision. Which fork in the road will you choose?

⬦⬦⬦⬦⬦⬦⬦⬦⬦⬦⬦⬦⬦⬦⬦⬦⬦⬦⬦⬦ **TODAY'S PRACTICE** ⬦⬦⬦⬦⬦⬦⬦⬦⬦⬦⬦⬦⬦⬦⬦⬦⬦⬦⬦⬦

Write about which fork in the road you will take and why that is your choice.

_____

_____

_____

_____

_____

_____

Your emotions and habits can impact the biology of your body so much that it can alter the genes you pass on to the next generation. Through the process of epigenetics, the impact of your diet, stress level, exposure to toxins, traumatic experiences, habits, and more can affect the genes that your children and grandchildren have.

When you choose to eat foods you love that love you back, take your daily supplements, manage your thoughts, reduce your BRIGHT MINDS risk factors, and regularly ask yourself, "Is this good for my brain or bad for it?," you increase the chances of passing along healthy genes. Every day of your life, you are also being a role model for the people in your life who matter to you. This is why brain health isn't just about you; it's about generations of you.

One of the most effective ways to keep this top-of-mind is by using what I call anchor images. Since 50% of the brain is dedicated to vision, having visual cues and reminders about why you want to have a healthy brain is a very effective way to help you stay on track.

To create your own set of anchor images, go through your photos and pull out the ones that instantly remind you of why you want to have a better brain. Who do you need to be healthy for? Who needs you to be the best version of yourself that you can be? Who needs you to be a positive role model?

Put your anchor images where you can see them every day to remind yourself why you care about having a healthy brain and a healthy life.

TODAY'S PRACTICE

- Look at your anchor images every day.
- Consider telling 2 or 3 people why you want to have a healthier brain and why you want them to join you in doing this.

You Did It! Now Keep It Up!

Congratulations on finishing the Change Your Brain Every Day 28-Day Quick-Start Guide! I am so glad you are on your way to making brain health a daily habit. But please don't stop now! As I mentioned throughout this guide, taking care of your brain is something you must think about every single day. As you continue practicing this, you will find that it gets easier and easier. Because, let's face it, being sick and unhealthy is much harder on you than consciously making good decisions that support the health of your brain and body.

I know you can keep it going, and in doing so, you are being a much-needed positive role model for your loved ones and the other people around you.

I will be cheering you on!

Daniel G. Amen, MD

ADDITIONAL RESOURCES

AMEN CLINICS

Memory problems, mental health issues, and cognitive decline can't wait. At Amen Clinics, we're here for you. We offer in-clinic brain scanning and appointments, as well as mental telehealth, clinical evaluations, and therapy for adults, teens, children, and couples. Find out more by speaking to a specialist today at 888-288-9834 or visit our website at amenclinics.com.

BRAINMD

Fuel your brain with high-quality, brain-directed nutraceuticals and other brain health products at BrainMD.com.